BOOK TITLE

# HEALTHY AGING

SUBTITLE: Providing advice on staying active, eating well, and maintaining overall health as people age.

AUTHOR'S NAME

**ERIC UROH**

# Dedication

To all those who believe that age is not a limitation but a canvas for embracing life's vibrant colors,
This eBook is dedicated to you.

May its words inspire you to nurture your body, mind, and spirit,
May you journey through the years with grace, resilience, and joy.

Here's to embracing the gift of aging,
And living each day with vitality, purpose, and gratitude.

This book is for you—
For your health, your happiness, and your journey towards healthy aging.

With love and best wishes,

ERIC UROH

# Table Of Contents

# Introduction:

*In today's world, the concept of aging has evolved beyond mere survival into a pursuit of vitality and well-being. "Healthy Aging" is not just about growing older; it's about embracing a lifestyle that nurtures physical, mental, and emotional health to ensure a fulfilling and enriching later life. This book is dedicated to guiding you on this journey toward optimal health and wellness as you age gracefully.*

A. **Definition of healthy aging**:

Healthy aging encompasses the process of maintaining and optimizing physical, mental, and social well-being as individuals grow older. It's about embracing the changes that come with age while proactively taking steps to preserve vitality, independence, and quality of life.

B. **Importance of maintaining health as people age**:

As we advance in years, the significance of prioritizing health becomes increasingly apparent. Aging is accompanied by a myriad of biological changes, health concerns, and life transitions that require careful attention and proactive management. By investing in our health and well-being, we not only enhance our longevity but also ensure that we can continue to lead active, fulfilling lives well into our later years.

C. **Overview of what the book will cover**:

This comprehensive guide to healthy aging explores a wide range of topics designed to empower you to take control of your health and embrace the aging process with confidence. From understanding the biological mechanisms of aging to practical strategies for staying active, eating well, and maintaining mental and emotional wellness, each chapter is packed with valuable insights, actionable tips, and evidence-based advice. Whether you're looking to enhance your fitness, optimize your nutrition, or navigate life's transitions with grace and resilience, this book provides the knowledge and tools you need to thrive at every stage of life.

As we embark on this journey together, let us embark with the understanding that aging is not a decline but an opportunity for growth, resilience, and profound self-discovery. Let us embrace the wisdom that comes with age and celebrate the richness of experience that makes each passing year a testament to the beauty and resilience of the human spirit.

# Chapter 1: Understanding Aging

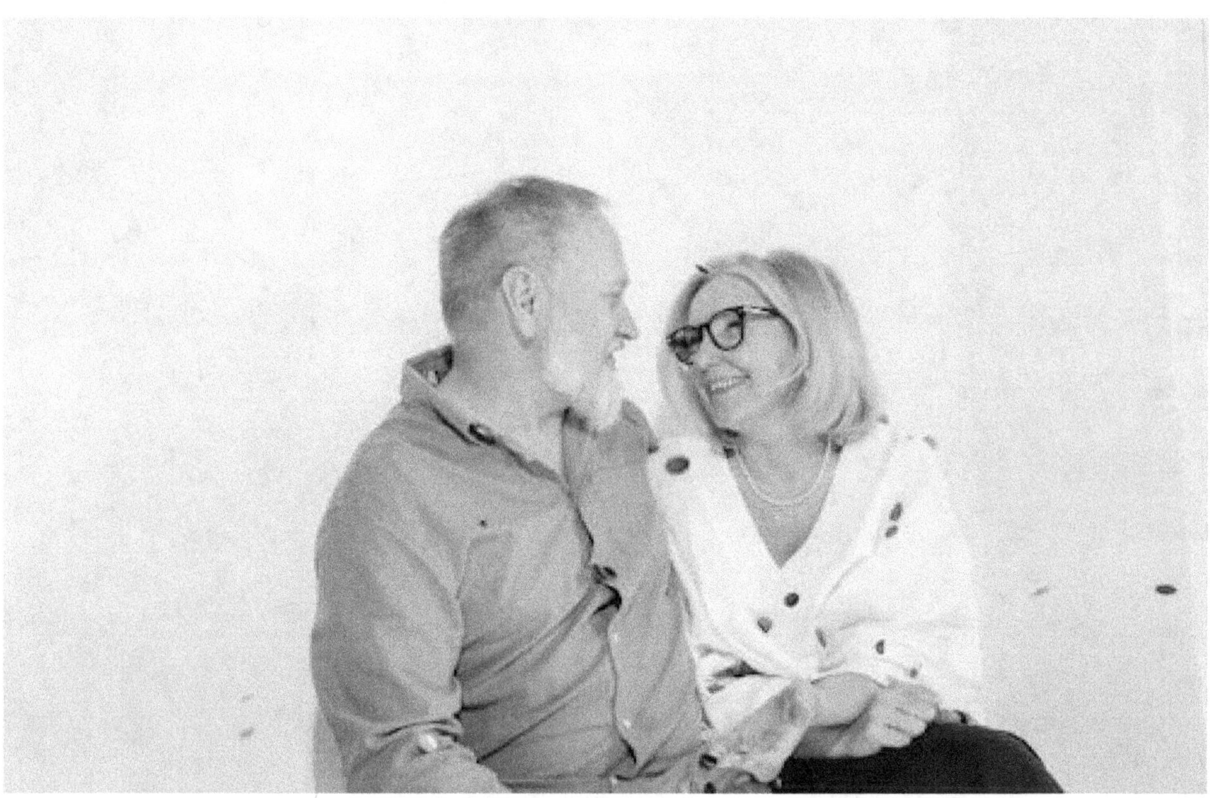

***A. Biological Changes that Occur with Aging:***

*As we journey through life, our bodies undergo a series of natural changes that are inherent to the aging process. These changes occur at the cellular, tissue, and organ levels, affecting various systems within the body. Some key biological changes associated with aging include:*

1. **Decline in Muscle Mass and Strength**: With advancing age, there is a gradual loss of muscle mass and strength, known as sarcopenia. This can lead to decreased mobility, balance issues, and an increased risk of falls.

2. **Reduction in Bone Density**: Aging is often accompanied by a decrease in bone density, leading to a higher susceptibility to fractures and osteoporosis, especially in postmenopausal women.

3. **Diminished Cardiovascular Function**: The cardiovascular system undergoes changes such as stiffening of blood vessels, decreased elasticity of the heart muscle, and changes in blood pressure regulation, which can contribute to an increased risk of heart disease and stroke.

4. **Decline in Immune Function**: The immune system undergoes alterations with age, resulting in decreased effectiveness in fighting off infections and an increased susceptibility to illnesses.

B. **Common Health Concerns Associated with Aging**:

While aging is a natural process, it is also associated with an increased risk of certain health concerns. Some common health issues that individuals may encounter as they age include:

1. **Chronic Diseases**: Conditions such as hypertension, diabetes, arthritis, and heart disease become more prevalent with age and require careful management to maintain health and well-being.

2. **Cognitive Decline**: Aging is often accompanied by changes in cognitive function, including memory loss, decreased processing speed, and an increased risk of neurodegenerative diseases such as Alzheimer's disease.

3. **Sensory Changes**: Vision and hearing may decline with age, leading to difficulties in seeing clearly or hearing conversations, which can impact daily functioning and quality of life.

4. **Mental Health Challenges**: Older adults may experience an increased risk of depression, anxiety, and other mental health disorders, often stemming from factors such as social isolation, loss of loved ones, or changes in life circumstances.

C. **Psychological Aspects of Aging**:

In addition to the physical changes that accompany aging, there are also important psychological dimensions to consider. Aging can bring about a range of emotional experiences and challenges, including:

1. **Adjusting to Life Transitions**: Retirement, changes in roles and responsibilities, and transitions in living arrangements can all impact one's sense of identity and purpose in later life.

2. **Coping with Loss and Grief**: As we age, we may experience the loss of friends, family members, or significant others, which can evoke feelings of grief, loneliness, and existential questioning.

3. **Maintaining Mental Resilience**: Cultivating resilience and coping skills is essential for navigating the inevitable challenges and stressors that come with aging, enabling individuals to adapt and thrive in the face of adversity.

By understanding the biological, health-related, and psychological aspects of aging, individuals can better prepare themselves to embrace the aging process with resilience, grace, and a proactive approach to maintaining their overall health and well-being.

# Chapter 2: Staying Active

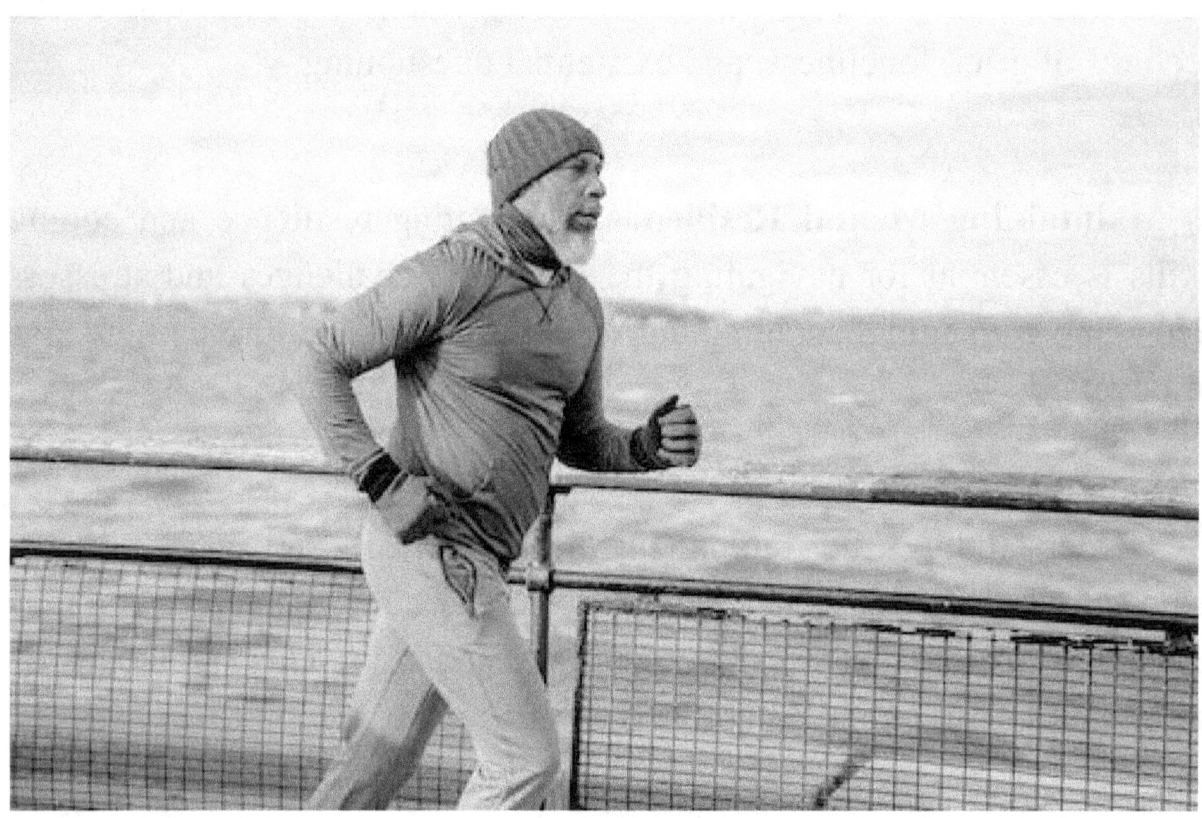

**A. Benefits of Physical Activity for Older Adults:**

*Physical activity is a cornerstone of healthy aging, offering a multitude of benefits for older adults. These include:*

1. **Improved Physical Health**: Regular exercise helps maintain muscle strength, flexibility, and bone density, reducing the risk of falls and fractures. It also enhances cardiovascular health, lowers blood pressure, and improves circulation.

2. **Enhanced Mental Well-being**: Exercise has been shown to reduce symptoms of depression and anxiety, enhance mood, and promote overall mental well-being. It can also improve cognitive function and lower the risk of cognitive decline and dementia.

3. **Increased Independence**: By improving strength, balance, and mobility, physical activity enables older adults to maintain their independence and perform daily activities with greater ease and confidence.

4. **Better Quality of Life**: Engaging in regular physical activity can enhance overall quality of life by promoting better sleep, increased energy levels, and a greater sense of vitality and self-esteem.

B. **Types of Exercises Suitable for Different Fitness Levels**:

It's essential for older adults to choose exercises that are appropriate for their fitness level and health status. Some examples of exercises suitable for different fitness levels include:

1. **Low-Impact Aerobic Activities**: Walking, swimming, cycling, and water aerobics are excellent options for older adults looking to improve cardiovascular health without placing excessive strain on joints.

2. **Strength Training**: Using resistance bands, free weights, or weight machines can help older adults build and maintain muscle mass, improve bone density, and prevent age-related muscle loss.

3. **Flexibility and Balance Exercises**: Yoga, tai chi, and gentle stretching routines help improve flexibility, balance, and coordination, reducing the risk of falls and enhancing overall mobility.

4. **Functional Exercises**: Functional exercises mimic activities of daily living and focus on movements such as bending, lifting, and reaching. These exercises help improve strength and mobility for performing everyday tasks more efficiently.

C. **Tips for Incorporating Physical Activity into Daily Routine**:

Incorporating physical activity into daily life doesn't have to be daunting. Here are some tips to help older adults make exercise a regular part of their routine:

1. **Start Slowly**: Begin with short, manageable sessions of physical activity and gradually increase duration and intensity as fitness improves.

2. **Find Activities You Enjoy**: Choose activities that you find enjoyable and fulfilling, whether they're dancing, gardening, or playing a sport. This increases the likelihood of sticking with it long term.

3. **Set Realistic Goals**: Set specific, achievable goals for your physical activity routine, such as walking for 30 minutes a day or completing a strength training session twice a week.

4. **Make It Social**: Exercise with friends, family members, or join group fitness classes to make physical activity more enjoyable and sociable.

D. **Overcoming Common Barriers to Exercise in Older Age**:

Despite the numerous benefits of exercise, older adults may encounter barriers that hinder their ability to stay active. Here are some strategies for overcoming common barriers:

1. **Addressing Pain and Injury**: Consult with a healthcare professional to address any pain or injury concerns and develop a safe and effective exercise plan tailored to your needs.

2. **Managing Chronic Conditions**: Work with your healthcare provider to manage chronic conditions such as arthritis, heart disease, or diabetes, and find exercises that are safe and appropriate for your condition.

3.  **Incorporating Adaptations**: Modify exercises as needed to accommodate physical limitations or health concerns, such as using assistive devices or opting for seated variations of exercises.

4. **Stay Motivated**: Find sources of motivation and support, whether it's setting goals, tracking progress, or seeking encouragement from friends and family.

By understanding the benefits of physical activity, choosing suitable exercises, incorporating activity into daily routines, and overcoming common barriers, older adults can enjoy improved health, vitality, and quality of life as they age.

17

# Chapter 3: Eating Well

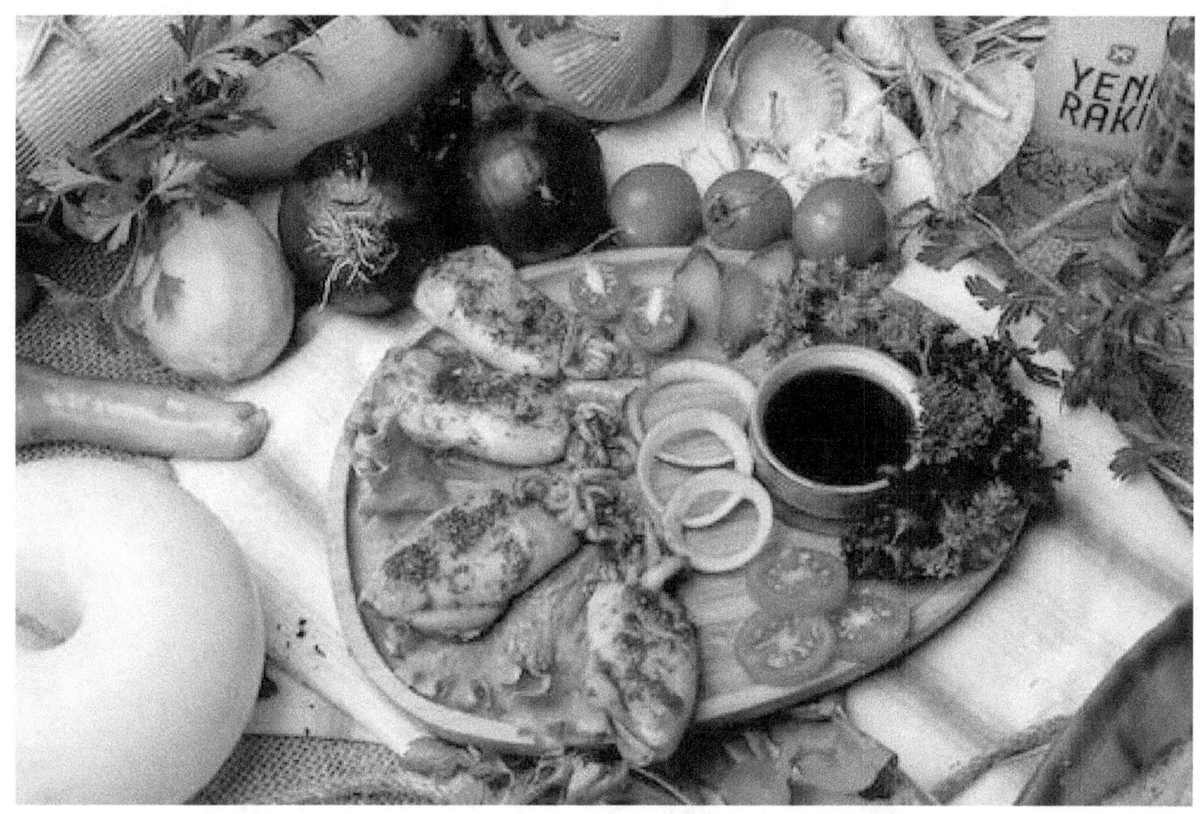

## *A. Importance of Nutrition for Healthy Aging:*

*Nutrition plays a crucial role in promoting healthy aging by providing essential nutrients that support overall well-being and help prevent age-related diseases. Proper nutrition is vital for:*

1. **Maintaining Muscle Mass and Strength**: Adequate protein intake is essential for preserving muscle mass and strength, which is particularly important for older adults to prevent sarcopenia and maintain mobility.

2. **Supporting Bone Health**: Calcium, vitamin D, and other nutrients found in a balanced diet are essential for maintaining bone density and reducing the risk of osteoporosis and fractures.

3. **Promoting Heart Health**: A diet rich in fruits, vegetables, whole grains, and healthy fats can help lower cholesterol levels, blood pressure, and inflammation, reducing the risk of heart disease and stroke.

4. **Enhancing Cognitive Function**: Certain nutrients, such as omega-3 fatty acids, antioxidants, and vitamins B6, B12, and folate, play a role in maintaining cognitive function and reducing the risk of cognitive decline and dementia.

B. **Nutritional Needs and Dietary Recommendations for Older Adults**:

As we age, our nutritional needs may change due to factors such as changes in metabolism, decreased appetite, and alterations in nutrient absorption. Key dietary recommendations for older adults include:

1. **Adequate Hydration**: Older adults may be at increased risk of dehydration due to decreased thirst sensation and changes in kidney function. Drinking plenty of fluids, including water, herbal tea, and low-sodium broth, is essential for maintaining hydration.

2. **Protein-Rich Foods**: Incorporating sources of high-quality protein, such as lean meats, poultry, fish, eggs, dairy products, legumes, and nuts, into meals and snacks helps support muscle health and repair.

3. **Fiber-Rich Foods**: Consuming a variety of fruits, vegetables, whole grains, beans, and legumes provides fiber, which aids in digestion, promotes regular bowel movements, and helps reduce the risk of constipation and diverticulosis.

4. **Nutrient-Dense Foods**: Focus on nutrient-dense foods that provide essential vitamins, minerals, and antioxidants while limiting empty calories from processed foods, sugary snacks, and high-fat desserts.

C. **Strategies for Meal Planning and Portion Control**:

Effective meal planning and portion control are essential for maintaining a healthy diet and managing weight as we age. Here are some strategies to help older adults plan nutritious meals and control portion sizes:

1. **Plan Balanced Meals**: Aim to include a variety of food groups in each meal, including lean proteins, whole grains, fruits, vegetables, and healthy fats, to ensure a well-rounded diet.

2. **Use Smaller Plates**: Opt for smaller plates and bowls to help control portion sizes and prevent overeating.

3. **Practice Mindful Eating**: Pay attention to hunger and fullness cues, eat slowly, and savor each bite to avoid overeating and promote satisfaction.

4. **Pre-Portion Snacks**: Portion out snacks into single servings to avoid mindless munching and help control calorie intake.

D. **Addressing Common Nutritional Challenges in Older Age**:

Older adults may face specific nutritional challenges that require attention and adaptation. Some common challenges include:

1. **Reduced Appetite**: Aging can lead to decreased appetite, which may result in inadequate nutrient intake. Eating smaller, more frequent meals and incorporating nutrient-dense snacks can help meet nutritional needs.

2. **Dental Problems**: Dental issues such as tooth decay, gum disease, and tooth loss can make chewing and swallowing difficult. Opting for soft, easy-to-chew foods and incorporating smoothies, soups, and pureed foods can help address these challenges.

3. **Medication Interactions**: Certain medications may affect appetite, nutrient absorption, or metabolism. It's essential to discuss any potential medication-nutrient interactions with a healthcare provider and adjust dietary intake accordingly.

4. **Digestive Issues**: Digestive issues such as constipation, acid reflux, and lactose intolerance may become more common with age. Consuming fiber-rich foods, staying hydrated, and avoiding trigger foods can help alleviate symptoms and promote digestive health.

By understanding the importance of nutrition for healthy aging, following dietary recommendations tailored to older adults, implementing strategies for meal planning and portion control, and addressing common nutritional challenges, older adults can support their overall health and well-being through proper nutrition.

# Chapter 4: Maintaining Mental and Emotional Health

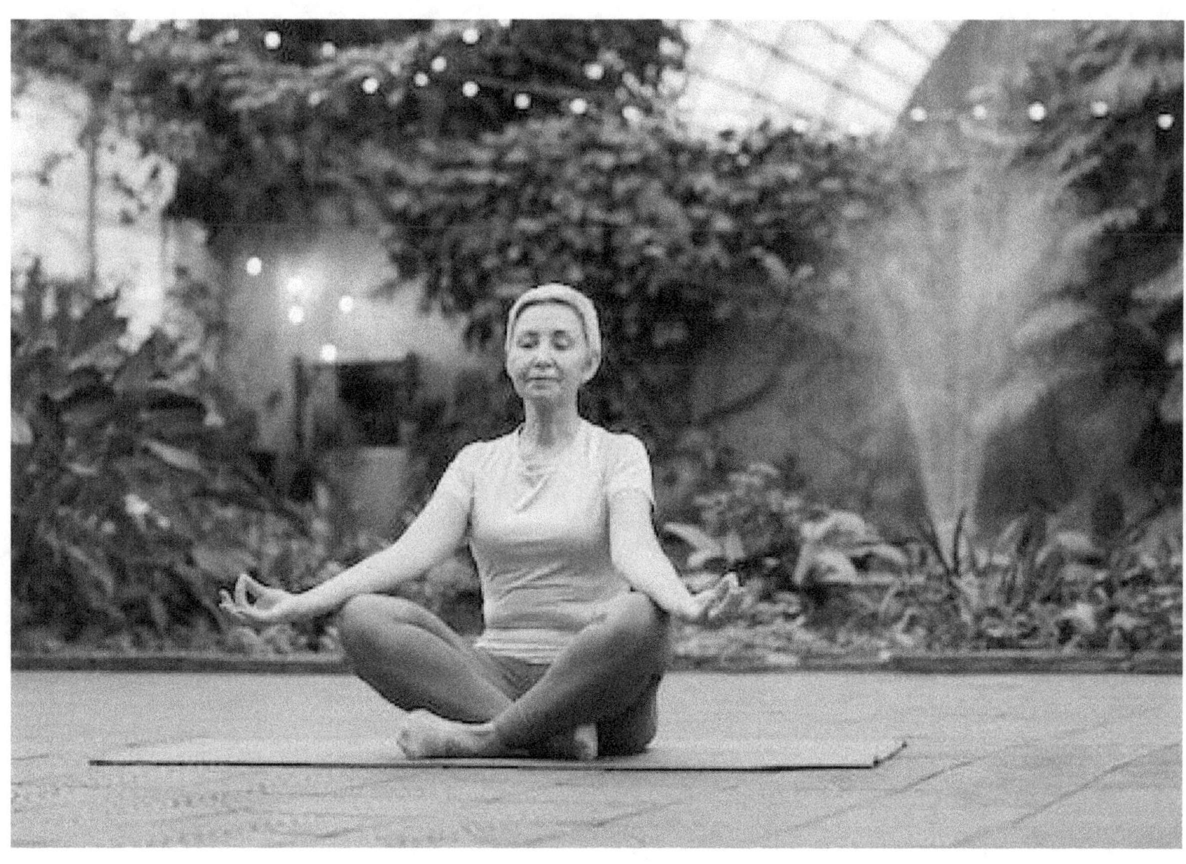

*A. Strategies for Reducing Stress and Anxiety:*

*Stress and anxiety can take a toll on mental and emotional well-being, especially as we age. Implementing effective strategies to manage stress and anxiety is essential for maintaining overall health and resilience. Some strategies to reduce stress and anxiety include:*

1. **Mindfulness and Meditation**: Practice mindfulness techniques such as deep breathing exercises, meditation, and progressive muscle relaxation to promote relaxation and reduce stress levels.

2. **Engage in Relaxation Activities**: Participate in activities that promote relaxation and stress relief, such as yoga, tai chi, gardening, or listening to calming music.

3. **Stay Active**: Regular physical activity has been shown to reduce stress and anxiety levels by releasing endorphins, the body's natural mood lifters. Aim for at least 30 minutes of moderate exercise most days of the week.

4. **Prioritize Self-Care**: Take time for self-care activities that nurture your mental and emotional well-being, such as reading, journaling, taking baths, or engaging in hobbies you enjoy.

B. **Importance of Social Connections and Staying Engaged**:

Maintaining social connections and staying engaged in meaningful activities are essential for promoting mental and emotional health as we age. Social interaction provides opportunities for companionship, support, and a sense of belonging. Ways to foster social connections and stay engaged include:

1. **Cultivate Relationships**: Stay connected with friends, family members, and community groups through regular phone calls, video chats, or in-person visits.

2. **Join Clubs or Groups**: Participate in clubs, classes, or hobby groups that align with your interests and passions, providing opportunities to meet new people and engage in enjoyable activities.

3. **Volunteer**: Volunteering can provide a sense of purpose, fulfillment, and social connection while giving back to the community. Look for volunteer opportunities in your area that match your skills and interests.

4. **Stay Active in Your Community**: Attend local events, cultural activities, or religious gatherings to stay connected with your community and engage in meaningful social interactions.

**C. Cognitive Exercises and Activities to Keep the Mind Sharp:**

Keeping the mind sharp and engaged is crucial for maintaining cognitive function and preventing cognitive decline as we age. Incorporate cognitive exercises and activities into your daily routine to challenge your brain and promote mental agility. Some activities to keep the mind sharp include:

1. **Puzzles and Brain Games**: Engage in activities such as crossword puzzles, Sudoku, brain teasers, or memory games to stimulate cognitive function and improve problem-solving skills.

2. **Learn Something New**: Take up a new hobby, learn a musical instrument, or enroll in classes or workshops to challenge your mind and expand your knowledge.

3. **Read and Write Regularly**: Reading books, newspapers, or magazines and writing in a journal or engaging in creative writing exercises can help maintain cognitive function and stimulate the brain.

4. **Stay Curious**: Cultivate a curious mindset by exploring new topics, asking questions, and seeking out new experiences to keep the brain active and engaged.

D. **Seeking Support for Mental Health Concerns**:

It's essential to seek support and professional help if you're experiencing mental health concerns such as depression, anxiety, or cognitive decline.

Don't hesitate to reach out to trusted friends, family members, or healthcare professionals for support and guidance. Some steps to take if you're struggling with mental health concerns include:

1. **Talk to Someone**: Share your feelings and concerns with someone you trust, whether it's a friend, family member, or mental health professional. Opening up about your struggles can help alleviate feelings of isolation and provide support.

2. **Seek Professional Help**: If you're experiencing persistent or severe mental health symptoms, consult with a mental health professional, such as a therapist, counselor, or psychiatrist, who can provide assessment, support, and treatment options.

3. **Explore Therapy Options**: Consider therapy or counseling as a way to explore your thoughts and feelings, learn coping skills, and develop strategies to manage mental health concerns effectively.

4. **Prioritize Self-Care**: Focus on self-care activities that promote mental and emotional well-being, such as getting adequate sleep, eating a balanced diet, exercising regularly, and practicing relaxation techniques.

By implementing strategies to reduce stress and anxiety, prioritizing social connections and engagement, engaging in cognitive exercises, and seeking support for mental health concerns, older adults can promote mental and emotional well-being and enjoy a fulfilling and meaningful life as they age.

# Chapter 5: Preventive Health Measures

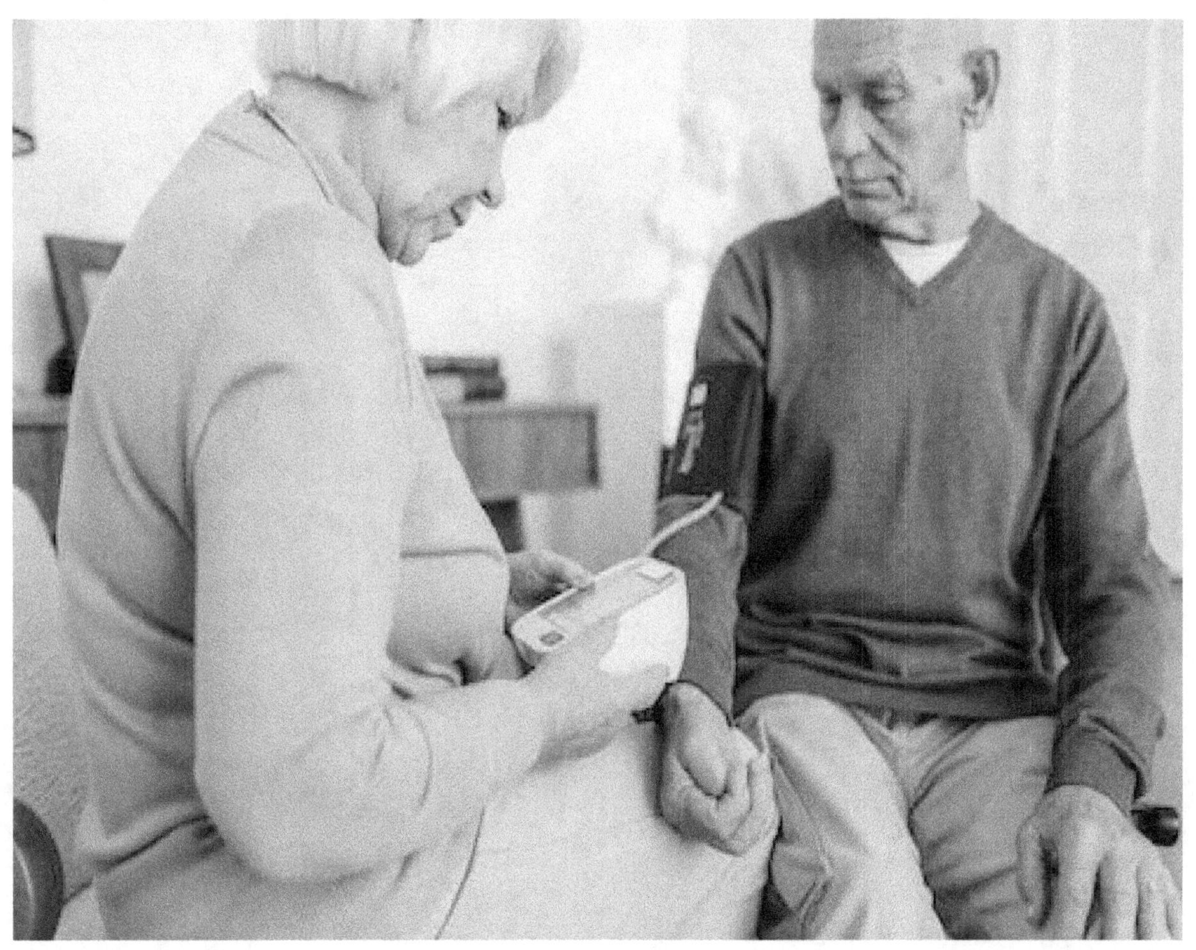

## *A. Importance of Regular Check-ups and Screenings:*

*Regular check-ups and screenings are crucial for maintaining optimal health and detecting potential health issues early, before they progress into more serious conditions. Some key reasons why regular check-ups and screenings are important for older adults include:*

1. **Early Detection of Health Issues**: Regular check-ups and screenings can help detect medical conditions such as high blood pressure, diabetes, cancer, and heart disease in their early stages when they are more treatable.

2. **Monitoring Chronic Conditions**: For individuals with chronic health conditions such as diabetes, hypertension, or arthritis, regular check-ups allow healthcare providers to monitor disease progression, adjust treatment plans as needed, and prevent complications.

3. **Preventive Care**: Check-ups also provide opportunities for preventive care, such as vaccinations, health screenings, and lifestyle counseling, which can help reduce the risk of developing certain diseases and promote overall well-being.

4. **Holistic Health Assessment**: Regular check-ups provide an opportunity for healthcare providers to assess not only physical health but also mental and emotional well-being, address concerns, and provide support and guidance for healthy aging.

B. **Vaccinations and Immunizations for Older Adults**:

Vaccinations and immunizations are essential for protecting older adults from infectious diseases and preventing serious complications. Some key vaccinations recommended for older adults include:

1. **Influenza (Flu) Vaccine**: The annual flu vaccine is recommended for all adults aged 65 and older to protect against seasonal influenza and its complications, which can be severe in older adults.

2. **Pneumococcal Vaccine**: The pneumococcal vaccine is recommended for adults aged 65 and older to protect against pneumococcal disease, including pneumonia, meningitis, and bloodstream infections.

3. **Shingles (Herpes Zoster) Vaccine**: The shingles vaccine is recommended for adults aged 50 and older to prevent shingles, a painful rash caused by the varicella-zoster virus.

4. **Other Vaccines**: Depending on individual health status and risk factors, older adults may also need vaccines such as the Tdap (tetanus, diphtheria, and pertussis) vaccine, hepatitis A and B vaccines, and the HPV vaccine.

C. **Managing Chronic Conditions and Medications Effectively**:

Managing chronic health conditions and medications effectively is essential for maintaining health and well-being as we age. Some strategies for managing chronic conditions and medications include:

1. **Regular Monitoring**: Work closely with healthcare providers to monitor chronic conditions through regular check-ups, screenings, and laboratory tests to ensure optimal disease management and prevent complications.

2. **Medication Management**: Keep an up-to-date list of all medications, including prescription drugs, over-the-counter medications, and supplements, and review it regularly with healthcare providers to prevent drug interactions, side effects, and medication errors.

3. **Adherence to Treatment Plans**: Follow prescribed treatment plans, including medication regimens, lifestyle modifications, and dietary recommendations, to effectively manage chronic conditions and optimize health outcomes.

4. **Communication with Healthcare Providers**: Maintain open and honest communication with healthcare providers, asking questions, expressing concerns, and seeking clarification about treatment plans, medications, and potential side effects.

D. **Tips for Promoting Good Sleep Hygiene**:

Good sleep hygiene is essential for overall health and well-being, especially as we age. Some tips for promoting good sleep hygiene include:

1. **Establish a Consistent Sleep Schedule**: Go to bed and wake up at the same time every day, even on weekends, to regulate your body's internal clock and promote restful sleep.

2. **Create a Relaxing Bedtime Routine**: Engage in calming activities before bed, such as reading, taking a warm bath, or practicing relaxation techniques, to signal to your body that it's time to wind down and prepare for sleep.

3. **Create a Comfortable Sleep Environment**: Make your bedroom conducive to sleep by keeping it dark, quiet, and cool, investing in a comfortable mattress and pillows, and minimizing distractions such as electronic devices.

4. **Limit Stimulants and Electronics Before Bed**: Avoid consuming caffeine, nicotine, and heavy meals close to bedtime, and limit exposure to electronic devices such as smartphones, computers, and televisions, which can interfere with sleep.

By prioritizing regular check-ups and screenings, staying up-to-date on vaccinations and immunizations, effectively managing chronic conditions and medications, and promoting good sleep hygiene, older adults can take proactive steps to maintain their health, prevent disease, and age gracefully.

# Chapter 6: Lifestyle Factors for Healthy Aging

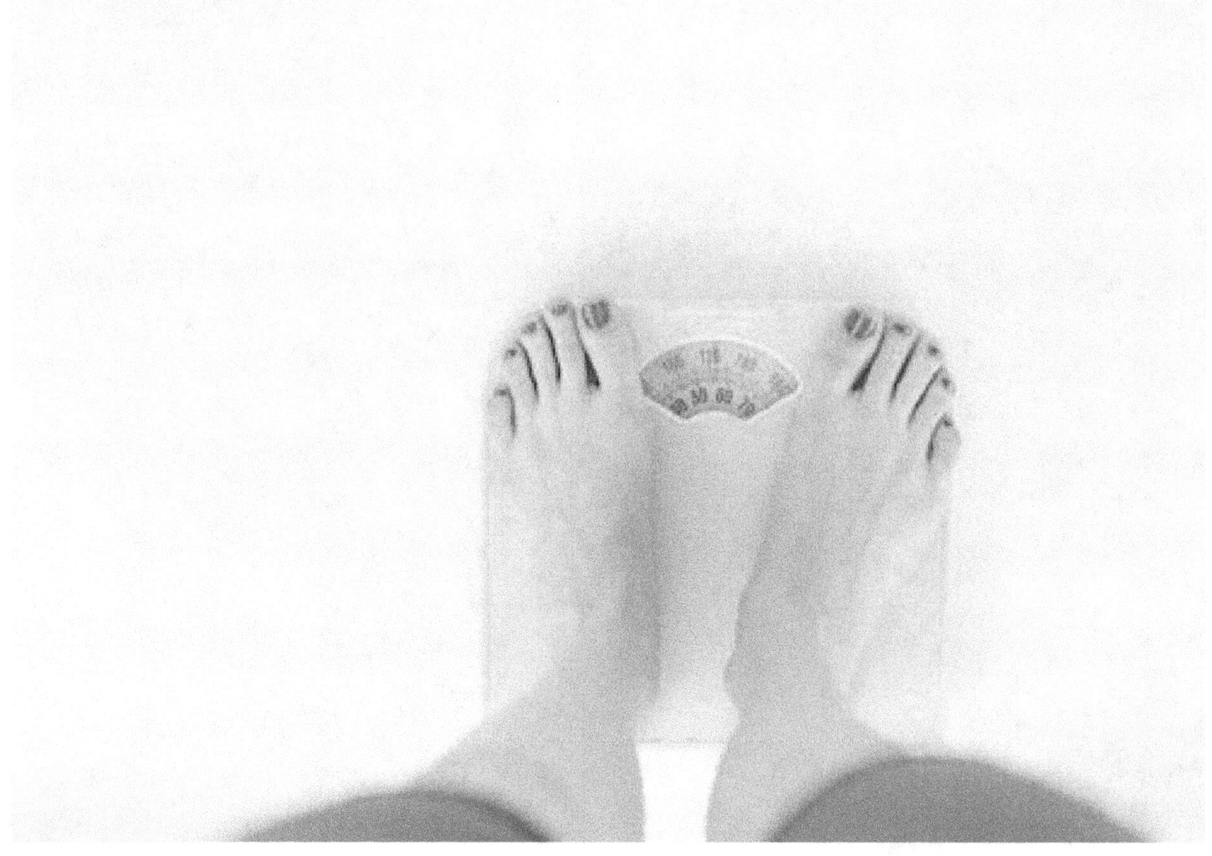

## *A. Importance of Maintaining a Healthy Weight:*

*Maintaining a healthy weight is crucial for overall health and well-being as we age. Excess weight, particularly around the abdomen, is associated with an increased risk of chronic diseases such as heart disease, diabetes, and certain cancers. Some reasons why maintaining a healthy weight is important for healthy aging include:*

1. **Reduced Risk of Chronic Diseases**: Maintaining a healthy weight can help reduce the risk of developing chronic conditions such as type 2 diabetes, hypertension, heart disease, stroke, and certain types of cancer.

2. **Improved Mobility and Function**: Excess weight can put strain on joints and muscles, leading to mobility issues and decreased physical function. Achieving and maintaining a healthy weight can improve mobility, flexibility, and overall physical function.

3. **Enhanced Quality of Life**: Maintaining a healthy weight can improve overall quality of life by increasing energy levels, reducing fatigue, and enhancing mood and self-esteem.

4. **Longevity**: Studies have shown that maintaining a healthy weight is associated with a longer life expectancy and a reduced risk of premature mortality.

B. **Managing Chronic Conditions such as Diabetes and Hypertension**:

Managing chronic conditions such as diabetes and hypertension is essential for promoting healthy aging and preventing complications. Some strategies for managing chronic conditions effectively include:

1. **Regular Monitoring**: Monitor blood sugar levels, blood pressure, and other relevant health markers regularly to track disease progression and make necessary adjustments to treatment plans.

2. **Medication Adherence**: Take prescribed medications as directed by healthcare providers to effectively manage chronic conditions and prevent complications.

3. **Lifestyle Modifications**: Adopt healthy lifestyle habits such as following a balanced diet, engaging in regular physical activity, managing stress, getting adequate sleep, and avoiding smoking and excessive alcohol consumption to help manage chronic conditions and improve overall health.

4. **Regular Follow-Up**: Schedule regular follow-up appointments with healthcare providers to monitor disease management, assess treatment effectiveness, and make any necessary adjustments to treatment plans.

C. **Limiting Alcohol Consumption and Avoiding Smoking**:

Limiting alcohol consumption and avoiding smoking are important lifestyle factors for promoting healthy aging and reducing the risk of chronic diseases and other health issues. Some reasons why limiting alcohol consumption and avoiding smoking are important include:

1. **Reduced Risk of Chronic Diseases**: Excessive alcohol consumption and smoking are both associated with an increased risk of chronic diseases such as heart disease, stroke, cancer, liver disease, and respiratory disorders.

2. **Improved Respiratory Health**: Smoking can damage the lungs and respiratory system, leading to conditions such as chronic obstructive pulmonary disease (COPD) and emphysema. Quitting smoking can improve respiratory health and reduce the risk of lung-related illnesses.

3. **Better Mental Health**: Excessive alcohol consumption and smoking are linked to mental health issues such as depression, anxiety, and cognitive decline. Limiting alcohol intake and avoiding smoking can help improve mental well-being and cognitive function.

4. **Longevity**: Studies have shown that reducing alcohol consumption and quitting smoking can increase life expectancy and improve overall health and well-being in older adults.

D. **Incorporating Relaxation Techniques and Hobbies for Stress Relief**:

Incorporating relaxation techniques and hobbies into daily life is essential for managing stress, promoting mental well-being, and enhancing overall quality of life. Some relaxation techniques and hobbies that can help relieve stress include:

1. **Mindfulness Meditation**: Practice mindfulness meditation to focus on the present moment, reduce stress and anxiety, and promote relaxation and inner peace.

2. **Deep Breathing Exercises**: Practice deep breathing exercises to activate the body's relaxation response, reduce stress levels, and promote calmness and relaxation.

3. **Engaging in Hobbies**: Engage in hobbies and activities that bring joy and fulfillment, such as gardening, painting, playing musical instruments, reading, cooking, or spending time in nature.

4. **Physical Activity**: Engage in regular physical activity such as walking, jogging, swimming, or yoga to reduce stress, improve mood, and promote overall well-being.

By prioritizing healthy lifestyle factors such as maintaining a healthy weight, managing chronic conditions effectively, limiting alcohol consumption and avoiding smoking, and incorporating relaxation techniques and hobbies for stress relief, older adults can promote healthy aging, enhance their quality of life, and enjoy a fulfilling and active lifestyle.

# Chapter 7: Adapting to Life Transitions

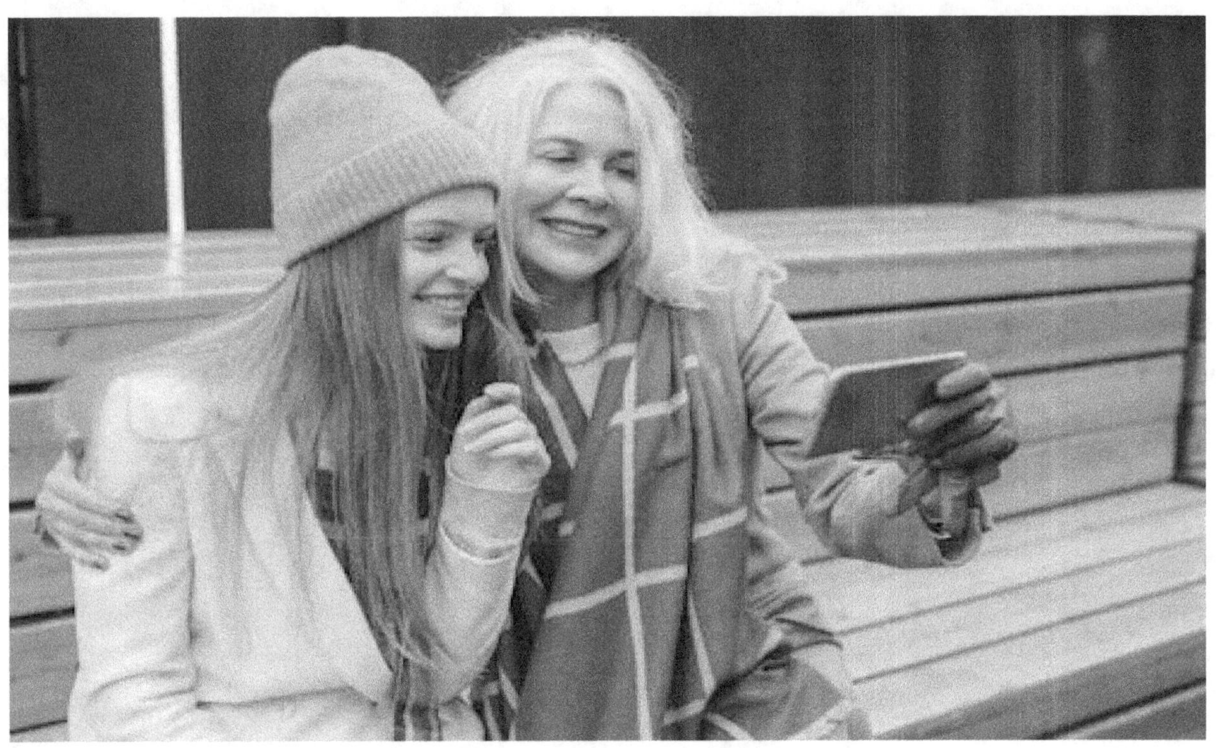

***A. Coping with Retirement and Changes in Routine:***

***Retirement marks a significant life transition that can bring about changes in routine, identity, and purpose. Coping with retirement effectively involves:***

1. **Establishing a New Routine**: Create a new daily schedule that includes activities you enjoy, such as hobbies, volunteering, or spending time with loved ones, to maintain a sense of structure and purpose.

2. **Exploring New Opportunities**: Embrace retirement as an opportunity to explore new interests, pursue lifelong dreams, or engage in activities that you didn't have time for during your working years.

3. **Seeking Social Support**: Lean on friends, family members, and support networks for emotional support and companionship during the transition to retirement. Joining clubs, groups, or community organizations can also provide opportunities for social connection and engagement.

4. **Reflecting on Accomplishments**: Take time to reflect on your accomplishments and achievements throughout your career and life, celebrating your successes and recognizing the contributions you've made.

**B. Adjusting to Physical Limitations and Mobility Challenges**:

As we age, we may encounter physical limitations and mobility challenges that require adaptation and adjustment. Some strategies for adjusting to physical limitations include:

1. **Seeking Assistive Devices**: Consider using assistive devices such as canes, walkers, or mobility aids to help maintain independence and mobility while navigating physical limitations.

2. **Modifying Living Spaces**: Make modifications to your home environment, such as installing grab bars, handrails, or ramps, to enhance safety and accessibility and accommodate physical limitations.

3. **Engaging in Physical Therapy**: Work with a physical therapist to develop a personalized exercise program that focuses on improving strength, flexibility, balance, and mobility, tailored to your individual needs and abilities.

4. **Embracing Adaptive Activities**: Explore adaptive sports, exercises, and activities that can be modified to accommodate physical limitations, such as chair yoga, water aerobics, or seated strength training.

C. **Finding Purpose and Meaning in Later Life**:

Finding purpose and meaning in later life is essential for maintaining mental and emotional well-being and enjoying a fulfilling and meaningful life. Some ways to find purpose and meaning include:

1. **Volunteering**: Volunteer for causes or organizations that align with your values and interests, providing opportunities to make a positive impact in your community and find fulfillment through service.

2. **Pursuing Passions**: Engage in activities, hobbies, or creative pursuits that bring you joy and fulfillment, whether it's painting, gardening, playing music, or writing.

3. **Mentoring and Teaching**: Share your knowledge, skills, and life experiences by mentoring others, volunteering as a tutor or coach, or teaching classes or workshops in your area of expertise.

4. **Connecting with Loved Ones**: Cultivate and strengthen relationships with family members, friends, and loved ones, nurturing meaningful connections and finding purpose in the bonds of love and companionship.

D. **Strategies for Maintaining Independence and Autonomy**:

Maintaining independence and autonomy is essential for promoting dignity, self-esteem, and quality of life as we age. Some strategies for maintaining independence include:

1. **Accessing Support Services**: Utilize support services and resources such as home care assistance, meal delivery programs, transportation services, and senior centers to help meet your needs while maintaining independence.

2. **Staying Active and Engaged**: Engage in physical, mental, and social activities that promote health, well-being, and independence, such as regular exercise, cognitive stimulation, and social engagement.

3. **Communicating Needs and Preferences**: Clearly communicate your needs, preferences, and wishes to family members, caregivers, and healthcare providers, advocating for yourself and actively participating in decision-making processes.

4. **Planning for the Future**: Take proactive steps to plan for the future, such as creating advance directives, establishing power of attorney, and making arrangements for long-term care, to maintain control over your decisions and affairs.

By adapting to life transitions, adjusting to physical limitations, finding purpose and meaning, and implementing strategies for maintaining independence and autonomy, older adults can navigate the aging process with resilience, grace, and a sense of purpose, enjoying a fulfilling and meaningful life in later years.

47

# Chapter 8: Planning for the Future

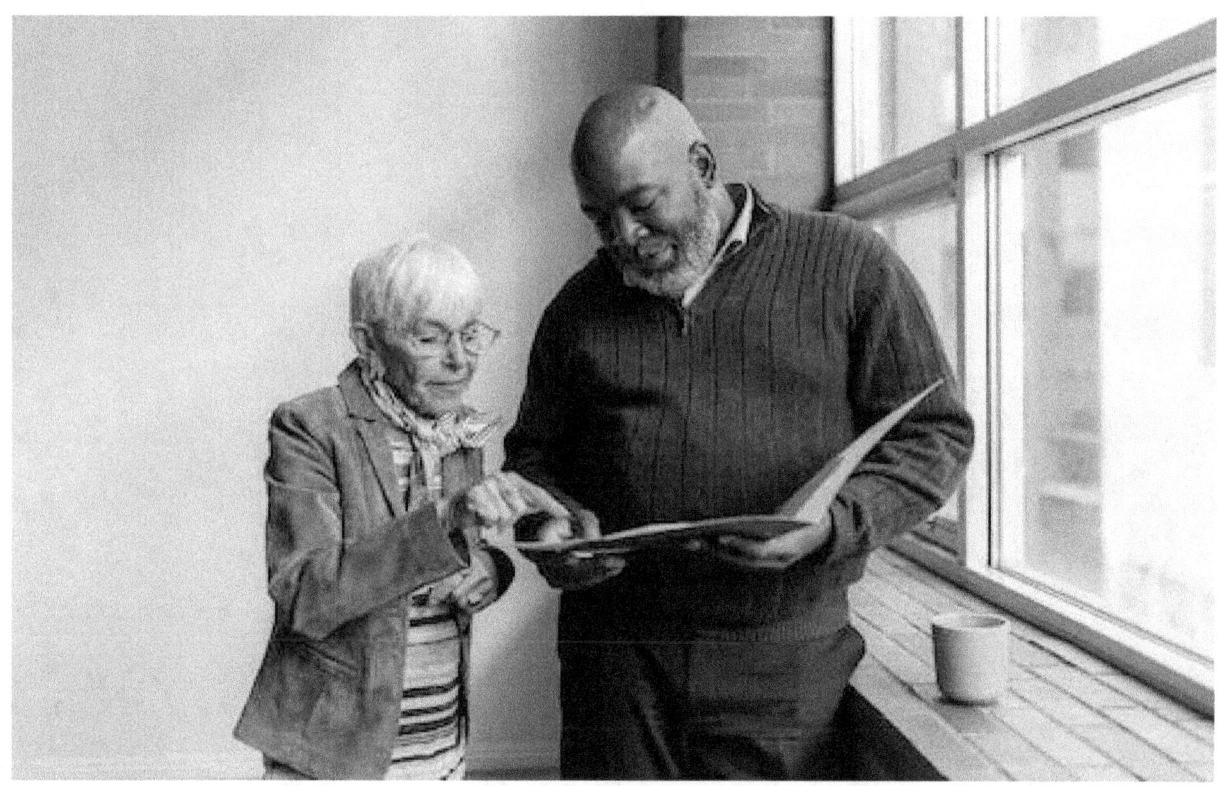

***A. Importance of Advance Care Planning and End-of-Life Decisions:***

*Advance care planning involves making decisions about future medical care and end-of-life preferences, ensuring that your wishes are known and respected in the event of incapacity or terminal illness. Some reasons why advance care planning is important include:*

1. **Ensuring Personal Preferences are Honored**: Advance care planning allows individuals to document their preferences for medical treatment, resuscitation, and end-of-life care, ensuring that healthcare decisions align with their values, beliefs, and wishes.

2. **Reducing Family Burden**: Having conversations about end-of-life preferences and documenting advance directives can alleviate the burden on family members and caregivers, who may otherwise struggle with difficult decisions during times of crisis.

3. **Facilitating Communication**: Advance care planning encourages open and honest communication between individuals, family members, and healthcare providers, promoting shared decision-making and clarity regarding medical wishes and goals of care.

4. **Providing Peace of Mind**: Engaging in advance care planning provides peace of mind, knowing that your preferences for medical care and end-of-life decisions are documented and will be respected, regardless of your ability to communicate them in the future.

B. **Financial Planning Considerations for Retirement and Long-Term Care**:

Financial planning is essential for ensuring a secure and comfortable future in retirement, including provisions for long-term care needs. Some key considerations for financial planning include:

1. **Retirement Savings**: Develop a comprehensive retirement savings plan, including contributions to retirement accounts such as 401(k)s, IRAs, or pension plans, to ensure financial security during retirement.

2. **Long-Term Care Insurance**: Consider purchasing long-term care insurance to cover the costs of assisted living, nursing home care, or in-home care services in the event of chronic illness or disability.

3. **Estate Planning**: Create a comprehensive estate plan that includes wills, trusts, and powers of attorney to protect assets, minimize estate taxes, and ensure that your wishes regarding inheritance and asset distribution are carried out.

4. **Budgeting and Financial Management**: Develop a budget and financial plan to manage expenses in retirement, including healthcare costs, housing expenses, and discretionary spending, to maintain financial stability and independence in later life.

C. **Resources for Accessing Support Services and Community Resources**:

Accessing support services and community resources can provide valuable assistance and assistance to older adults as they navigate the challenges of aging. Some resources to consider include:

1. **Area Agencies on Aging**: Area Agencies on Aging (AAA) provide a range of services and programs for older adults, including information and referral services, caregiver support, and assistance with accessing benefits and resources.

2. **Senior Centers**: Senior centers offer a variety of programs and activities for older adults, including social events, educational workshops, fitness classes, and support groups, providing opportunities for socialization and engagement.

3. **Caregiver Support Services**: Caregiver support services offer assistance and resources for family caregivers, including respite care, support groups, counseling, and educational programs to help caregivers navigate their caregiving role effectively.

4. **Community-Based Organizations**: Community-based organizations, such as religious institutions, nonprofit organizations, and civic groups, may offer services and programs tailored to the needs of older adults, such as transportation services, meal programs, and volunteer opportunities.

D. **Creating a Support Network and Communicating Wishes with Loved Ones**:

Creating a support network and communicating wishes with loved ones are essential aspects of planning for the future and ensuring that one's needs and preferences are known and respected. Some strategies for creating a support network and communicating wishes include:

1. **Identifying Trusted Individuals**: Identify trusted family members, friends, or professionals who can serve as advocates and provide support in making decisions regarding medical care, financial matters, and personal affairs.

2. **Having Conversations**: Initiate conversations with loved ones about your wishes for medical care, end-of-life preferences, and other important decisions, ensuring that your preferences are understood and respected.

3. **Documenting Advance Directives**: Complete advance directives, such as living wills, healthcare proxies, and durable powers of attorney for healthcare, to formally document your preferences for medical treatment and designate a trusted individual to make healthcare decisions on your behalf if you become incapacitated.

4. **Reviewing and Updating Plans**: Regularly review and update advance care plans, financial documents, and estate plans to reflect changes in preferences, circumstances, or relationships, ensuring that plans remain current and aligned with your wishes.

By engaging in advance care planning, addressing financial considerations, accessing support services and resources, and communicating wishes with loved ones, older adults can plan for the future with confidence, ensuring that their needs and preferences are known and respected as they age.

# Conclusion: Embracing Healthy Aging

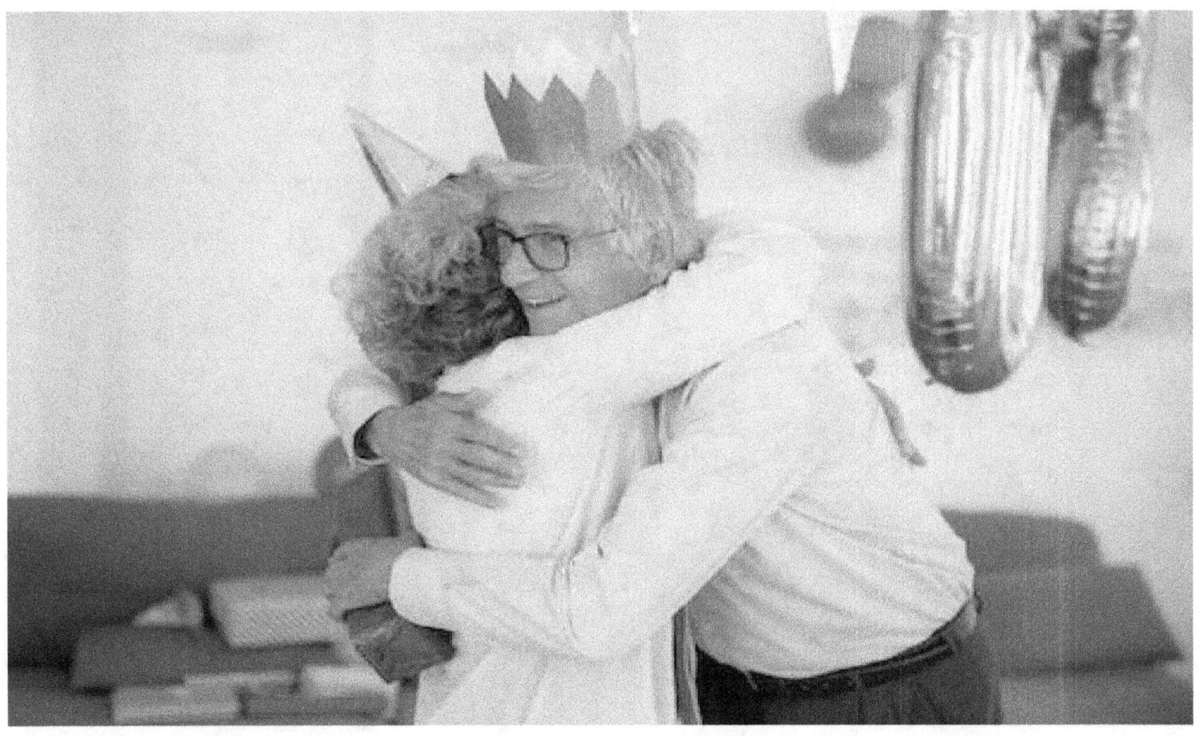

*As we conclude this journey through the intricacies of healthy aging, let us reflect on the key points that can guide us toward a vibrant and fulfilling life in our later years.*

## A. **Recap of Key Points for Healthy Aging**:

Throughout this book, we have explored various aspects of healthy aging, from physical well-being to mental resilience. We have learned the importance of:

- Prioritizing physical activity to maintain strength, flexibility, and overall health.

- Nourishing our bodies with nutritious foods to support vital functions and ward off disease.

- Cultivating mental and emotional well-being through stress management, social connections, and cognitive engagement.

- Taking preventive measures, such as regular check-ups, vaccinations, and screenings, to detect and manage health conditions.

- Embracing lifestyle factors like maintaining a healthy weight, managing chronic conditions, and avoiding harmful habits.

- Adapting to life transitions with grace, finding purpose and meaning in later life, and fostering independence and autonomy.

- Planning for the future by addressing advance care directives, financial considerations, and support networks.

## B. **Encouragement for Readers to Take Proactive Steps Towards Their Health**:

As we navigate the journey of aging, it's essential to remember that we hold the power to shape our health and well-being. By taking proactive steps toward our health, we can enhance our quality of life and embrace the aging process with resilience and vitality. Let us commit to:

- Prioritizing self-care and making healthy lifestyle choices that support our physical, mental, and emotional well-being.

- Advocating for ourselves by seeking regular medical check-ups, adhering to treatment plans, and advocating for our preferences in healthcare decisions.

- Cultivating meaningful relationships, engaging in fulfilling activities, and nurturing our passions and interests.

- Embracing change with openness and adaptability, recognizing that each stage of life brings new opportunities for growth and fulfillment.

**C. Final Thoughts on Embracing Aging as a Positive and Fulfilling Stage of Life:**

As we age, let us embrace the journey with gratitude, resilience, and a sense of purpose. Aging is not a decline but a continuation of life's journey—a journey enriched by wisdom, experience, and the profound beauty of each passing year. Let us celebrate the richness of life in all its stages, finding joy in the present moment and hope for the future.

In closing, remember that healthy aging is not merely the absence of illness but the presence of vitality, purpose, and fulfillment. May this book serve as a guide and inspiration as you embark on your own journey of healthy aging, embracing each day with gratitude, vitality, and the joy of living well.

Here's to a life of health, happiness, and flourishing at every age. Cheers to healthy aging!

# About The Author

Eric Uroh is a passionate advocate for health and well-being. With a deep concern for the overall wellness of individuals, Eric has dedicated his life to helping others achieve their health goals and lead happier, more fulfilling lives.

As a fervent fitness enthusiast, Eric Uroh brings a wealth of personal experience and knowledge to the realm of weight loss and healthy living. They have spent countless hours researching, experimenting with various strategies, and engaging in physical activities to discover what truly works for achieving and maintaining a healthy weight. This firsthand experience has given Eric Uroh unique insights into the challenges and triumphs that individuals face on their weight loss journeys.

Eric's unwavering commitment to health and well-being shines through in their writing, coaching, and advocacy work. They believe that everyone has the potential to transform their lives through informed choices and dedicated effort. Through this book, Eric shares his expertise, offering readers a practical and comprehensive guide to achieving their weight loss goals and embracing a healthier and happier lifestyle.

Join Eric Uroh on this transformative journey toward better health and discover the strategies and inspiration you need to embark on your own path to success. Your goals are within reach, and Eric is here to guide you every step of the way.

# Books By This Author

**Title: Fitness Motivation and Goal Setting**

**Description**:

Your Comprehensive Guide to Achieving Lasting Results and Transforming Your Life

Are you ready to embark on a transformative journey towards a healthier, stronger, and more vibrant you? "Fitness Motivation and Goal Setting" is your comprehensive guide to unlocking your full potential for lifelong health and wellness.

This eBook is your trusted companion on the path to fitness success, offering a roadmap that combines the power of motivation and effective goal setting. Inside, you'll discover the secrets to igniting and sustaining your motivation, setting smart and achievable fitness goals, and crafting a personalized fitness plan tailored to your unique needs and aspirations.

With practical insights, expert advice, and real-life success stories, you'll explore the art of overcoming obstacles, building resilience, and staying motivated throughout your journey. Dive into motivational techniques, harness the power of visualization, and learn the importance of accountability and support systems that will keep you on track.

As you progress through the chapters, you'll find inspiration in the stories of individuals who have already achieved remarkable fitness transformations. Discover the strategies that worked for them and apply these lessons to your own journey.

To equip you further, we've curated a valuable toolkit of resources and tools, including recommended apps, websites, fitness-tracking tools, books, podcasts, and online communities, ensuring you have the support you need every step of the way.

Your fitness journey is a lifelong adventure, and "Fitness Motivation and Goal Setting" is your trusted guide. Whether you're just starting or looking to revitalize your fitness routine, this eBook will empower you to set and achieve your goals, maintain momentum, and embrace a healthier, more fulfilling life. Begin your journey today and unlock the boundless potential within you. Your transformation starts now.

**Title: Weight Loss Strategies**

**Description**:

Unlock the Secrets to Sustainable Weight Loss and a Healthier You!

Are you tired of fad diets and quick fixes that don't deliver lasting results? Are you looking for a comprehensive guide to achieving your weight loss goals while improving your overall well-being? Look no further! "Weight Loss Strategies" is your ultimate resource for embarking on a transformative journey to a healthier and happier life.

Inside this eBook, you'll discover a wealth of knowledge and practical strategies that will empower you to take control of your weight and achieve sustainable results. Say goodbye to the cycle of yo-yo dieting and hello to a balanced, healthier lifestyle.

Here's what you can expect to find within these pages:

- The Science Behind Weight Loss: Understand the fundamentals of weight loss, from caloric deficits to metabolism and body composition. Gain the knowledge you need to make informed choices.

- Nutrition and Diet: Learn the art of healthy eating with insights into balanced diets, portion control, and mindful eating. Explore effective dietary plans, including low-carb diets, the Mediterranean diet, and intermittent fasting.

- Exercise and Physical Activity: Discover the importance of exercise in weight loss and explore various types of physical activities, from cardiovascular workouts to strength training and flexibility exercises. Create a personalized workout plan and learn how to stay consistent with your exercise routines.

- Lifestyle and Behavior Modification: Cultivate healthy habits for weight loss success, including the importance of sleep, stress management, and hydration. Break bad habits such as smoking and excessive alcohol consumption, and build a supportive environment with the help of family and friends or accountability partners.

- Monitoring and Tracking Progress: Unlock the power of progress tracking with insights into why it's crucial to monitor your weight and measurements. Keep a food journal, utilize technology and apps, and adjust your strategies based on your results.

- Dealing with Plateaus and Setbacks: Overcome common hurdles like weight loss plateaus with effective strategies. Learn how to handle setbacks and relapses while maintaining unwavering motivation during challenging times.

- Weight Maintenance: Successfully transition from weight loss to maintenance, develop a sustainable lifestyle, prevent weight regain, and celebrate your achievements and milestones.

In "Weight Loss Strategies," you'll find evidence-based guidance, practical tips, and expert advice to help you navigate the complexities of weight loss. Whether you're a beginner just starting your journey or someone looking to refine their approach, this eBook is your comprehensive roadmap to a healthier, happier life.

Don't wait any longer to take control of your weight and well-being. Get started on your path to success with "Weight Loss Strategies" today! Your transformation begins here.

**Title: Healthy Cooking**

**Description**:

Are you ready to embark on a culinary journey that will transform the way you approach food and nourish your body? "Healthy Cooking 101" is your comprehensive guide to a more vibrant, balanced, and health-conscious lifestyle through the art of cooking.

In this thoughtfully crafted eBook, you will explore the fundamental principles of healthy cooking, from understanding nutritional basics to mastering cooking techniques that preserve nutrients and enhance flavors. Discover how to plan well-balanced meals that incorporate lean proteins, whole grains, and an abundance of vegetables and fruits.

"Healthy Cooking" caters to a wide range of dietary needs and preferences, offering guidance on weight management, heart health, diabetes management, allergies, sensitivities, and even vegetarian and vegan cooking. With a focus on quality ingredients, you'll learn how to create delicious and nutritious recipes for breakfast, lunch, dinner, snacks, desserts, and beverages.

But this eBook goes beyond the kitchen. It delves into the holistic aspects of healthy living, helping you integrate exercise, manage stress, and make ethical food choices that align with your values. Explore how mindful eating and social connections enrich your relationship with food.

As you journey through the pages of "Healthy Cooking," you'll gain valuable insights into overcoming common challenges, staying on track with your goals, seeking support and accountability, and celebrating your successes.

Whether you're a seasoned home cook or just beginning to explore the joys of the kitchen, this eBook provides you with the knowledge, inspiration, and practical tools to make healthy cooking a sustainable and rewarding part of your life. Take the first step toward a healthier, happier you and embark on a culinary adventure that nourishes both body and soul. Your future of flavorful, nutritious meals starts here.

**Title: Fitness for Busy Professionals**

**Description:**

In the fast-paced world of modern professionals, finding time for fitness amidst the demands of a career can seem like an insurmountable challenge. Yet, maintaining a healthy lifestyle is essential for thriving in both personal and professional spheres. "Fitness for Busy Professionals" is a comprehensive guide tailored specifically for individuals navigating the intricate balance between career ambitions and well-being.

This eBook delves into the unique challenges faced by busy professionals, from time constraints and mental exhaustion to sedentary lifestyles and limited resources. It offers practical strategies and time-saving tips for integrating fitness into even the busiest of schedules, empowering readers to prioritize their health without sacrificing professional success.

From mindful scheduling and micro-workouts to leveraging technology and incorporating stress management techniques, this eBook provides actionable insights to help busy professionals overcome obstacles and establish sustainable fitness routines. Each chapter is packed with valuable information, actionable steps, and real-world examples to guide readers on their journey to improved health and vitality.

With a focus on cultivating a positive mindset, setting realistic goals, and celebrating progress, "Fitness for Busy Professionals" equips readers with the tools and motivation needed to make lasting lifestyle changes. It emphasizes the importance of self-care, encourages individuals to prioritize their well-being amidst career demands, and empowers them to take control of their health journey.

Whether you're a CEO with a packed schedule or an entrepreneur juggling multiple projects, this eBook is your roadmap to achieving fitness success during a hectic professional life. Let "Fitness for Busy Professionals" be your guide as you embark on a journey towards improved health, increased energy, and enhanced productivity. It's time to invest in yourself and unlock your full potential because a healthier, happier you is the key to thriving in every aspect of your life.

**Title: Fitness for Busy Professionals**

**Description:**

In the fast-paced world of modern professionals, finding time for fitness amidst the demands of a career can seem like an insurmountable challenge. Yet, maintaining a healthy lifestyle is essential for thriving in both personal and professional spheres. "Fitness for Busy Professionals" is a comprehensive guide tailored specifically for individuals navigating the intricate balance between career ambitions and well-being.

This eBook delves into the unique challenges faced by busy professionals, from time constraints and mental exhaustion to sedentary lifestyles and limited resources. It offers practical strategies and time-saving tips for integrating fitness into even the busiest of schedules, empowering readers to prioritize their health without sacrificing professional success.

From mindful scheduling and micro-workouts to leveraging technology and incorporating stress management techniques, this eBook provides actionable insights to help busy professionals overcome obstacles and establish sustainable fitness routines. Each chapter is packed with valuable information, actionable steps, and real-world examples to guide readers on their journey to improved health and vitality.

With a focus on cultivating a positive mindset, setting realistic goals, and celebrating progress, "Fitness for Busy Professionals" equips readers with the tools and motivation needed to make lasting lifestyle changes. It emphasizes the importance of self-care, encourages individuals to prioritize their well-being amidst career demands, and empowers them to take control of their health journey.

Whether you're a CEO with a packed schedule or an entrepreneur juggling multiple projects, this eBook is your roadmap to achieving fitness success during a hectic professional life. Let "Fitness for Busy Professionals" be your guide as you embark on a journey towards improved health, increased energy, and enhanced productivity. It's time to invest in yourself and unlock your full potential because a healthier, happier you is the key to thriving in every aspect of your life.